Neuroanatomy
COLORING BOOK
2nd Edition

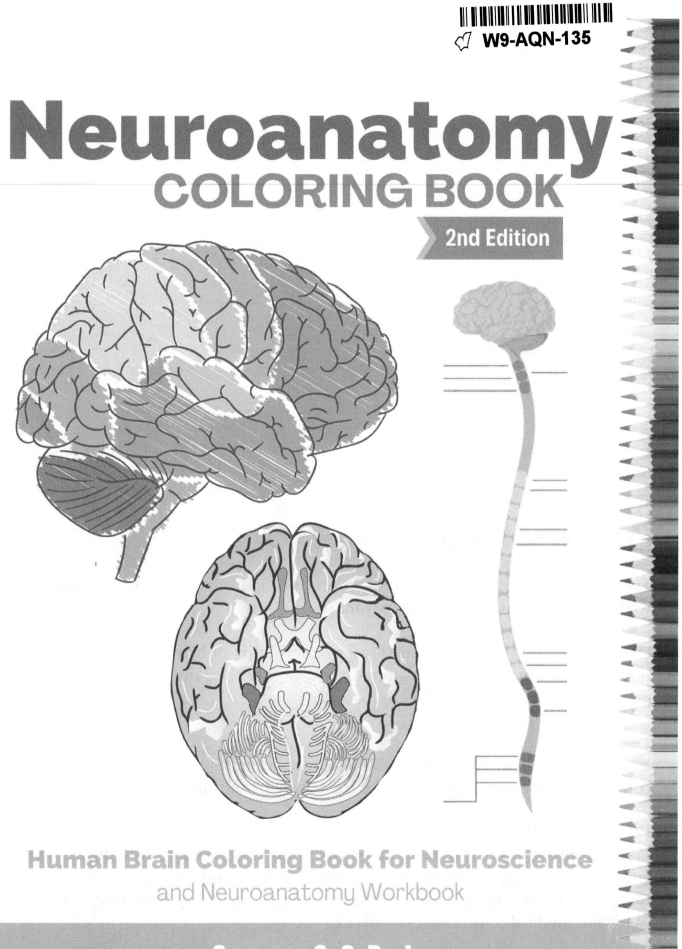

Human Brain Coloring Book for Neuroscience
and Neuroanatomy Workbook

Summer Q. S. Parks

INTRODUCTION

This book is an introduction to neuroanatomy, and my goal is to help you become familiar with the correct anatomical terms and be able to locate them by coloring them.

Ideal for those who want to increase their knowledge about the components, structure and functions of the nervous system and the brain. It is a book for all ages.

I hope you thoroughly enjoy it!

TABLE OF CONTENTS

Brain Anatomy

TABLE OF CONTENTS

TABLE OF CONTENTS

Neurons

Conclusion

BRAIN ANATOMY

The **brain** is an important part of the human body, and is protected by the skull and cerebrospinal fluid. This organ helps to rule all body functions, convert information from external signals, initiate body movement and control behavior.

Color the name and the labeled part:

Lateral View

1. Frontal Lobe
2. Temporal Lobe
3. Parietal Lobe
4. Occipital Lobe

Dorsal View

5. Frontal Lobe
6. Parietal Lobe
7. Occipital Lobe

The **brain** is divided into lobes, and each hemisphere has 4 lobes with different and specific functions: frontal, temporal, parietal, and occipital (*functions are detailed later in this book*).

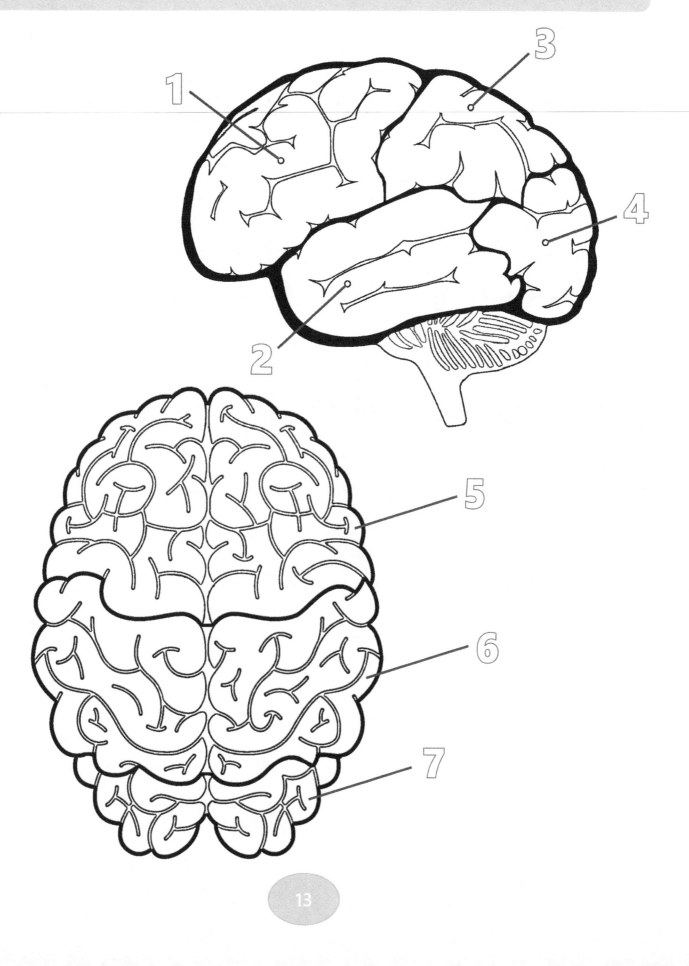

Color the name and the labeled part:

1. Superior frontal gyrus
2. Middle frontal gyrus
3. Inferior frontal gyrus
4. Supramarginal gyrus
5. Angular gyrus
6. Occipital gyrus
7. Precentral sulcus
8. Precentral gyrus
9. Central sulcus
10. Postcentral gyrus
11. Postcentral sulcus

Gyri are the folds in the brain, and sulci are the indentations in the brain, that give it its unique appearance.

Gyri and Sulci of the Brain (Dorsal View)

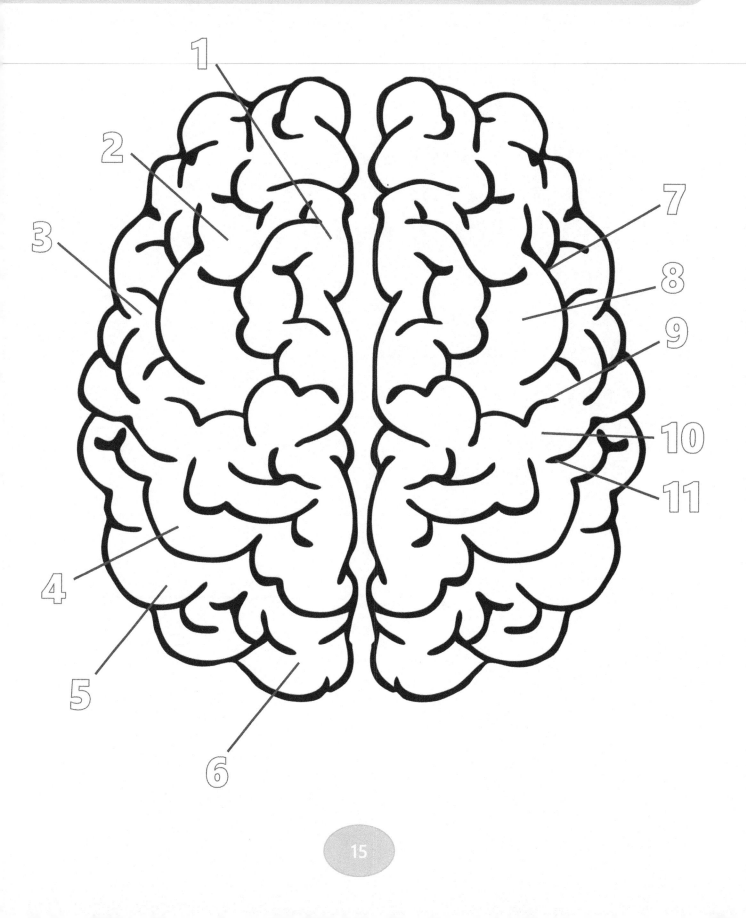

1

2

3

4

5

6

7

8

9

10

11

Color the name and the labeled part:

1. Orbital Sulcus
2. Orbital Gyrus
3. Inferior Temporal Sulcus
4. Inferior Temporal Gyrus
5. Longitudinal cerebral fissure
6. Olfactory Bulb
7. Optic chiasm
8. Mammillary Body
9. Pons
10. Medulla
11. Cerebellum

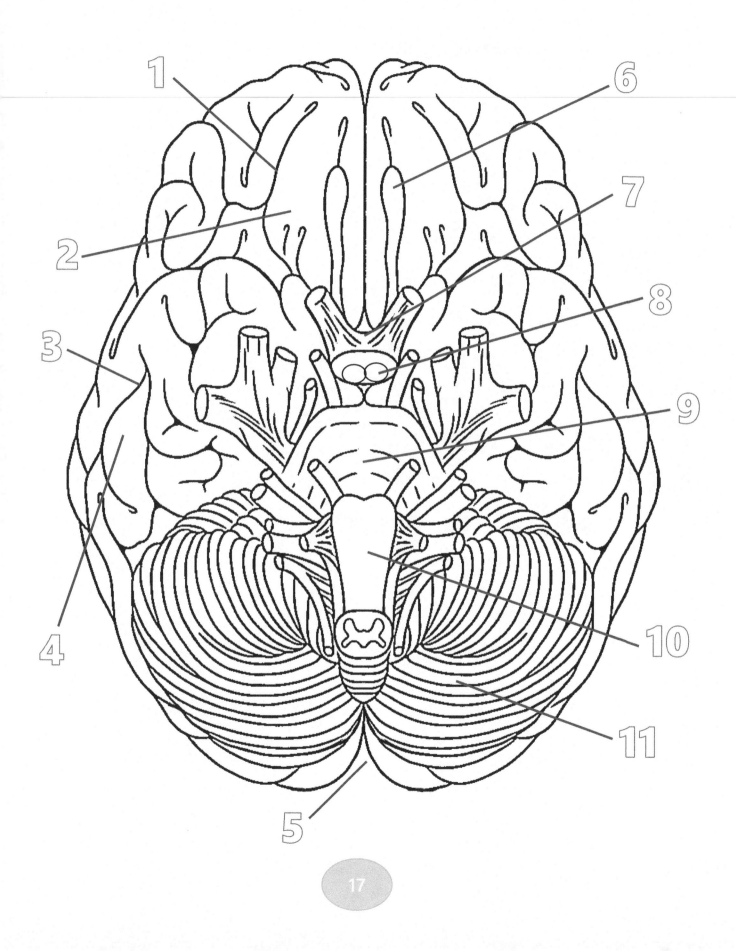

1

6

2

7

3

8

9

4

10

5

11

Color the name and the labeled part:

1. Frontal Lobe
2. Hypothalamus
3. Optic chiasm
4. Corpus callosum
5. Thalamus
6. Pineal gland
7. Fourth ventricle
8. Pituitary gland
9. Mammillary body
10. Pons
11. Medulla oblongata
12. Cerebellum

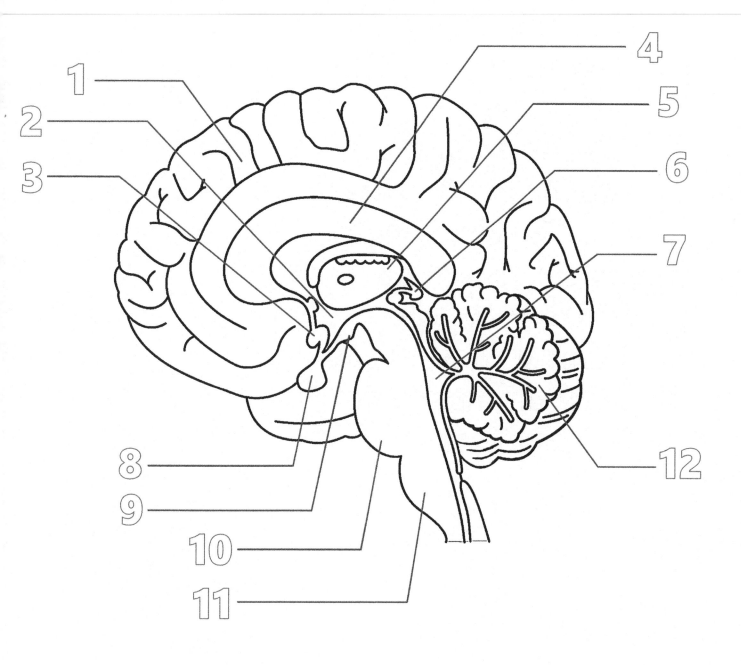

1

2

3

4

5

6

7

8

9

10

11

12

Color the name and the labeled part:

1. Caudate nucleus
2. Thalamus
3. Putamen
4. Globus pallidus
5. Subthalamic nucleus
6. Substantia nigra
7. Cerebral cortex
8. Third ventricle
9. Longitudinal fissure
10. Lateral ventricle
11. Lateral fissure

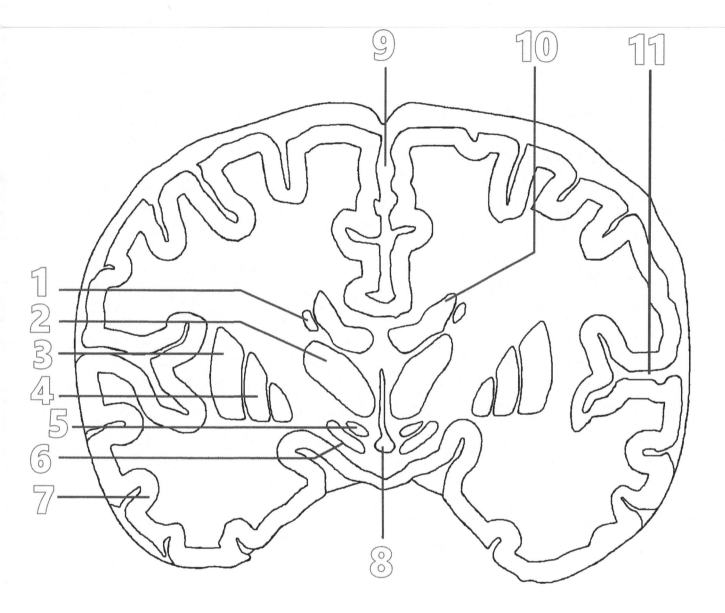

9

10

11

1

2

3

4

5

6

7

8

Color the name and the labeled part:

1. Ventral column
2. Ventral horn
3. Lateral column
4. Dorsal horn
5. Dorsal columns
6. Spinal canal
7. Lateral horn
8. Dorsal root filaments
9. Dorsal root
10. Dorsal root ganglion
11. Spinal nerve

12. Ventral root
13. Ventral root filaments
14. Spinal pia matter
15. Subarachnoid space
16. Spinal arachnoid
17. Spinal dura mater

The **spinal cord** is a cylindrical and long bundle of nervous tissue that extends from the brainstem to the lumbar vertebra. It is protected by the following layers of meninges: the pia mater, the dura mater and the arachnoid mater.

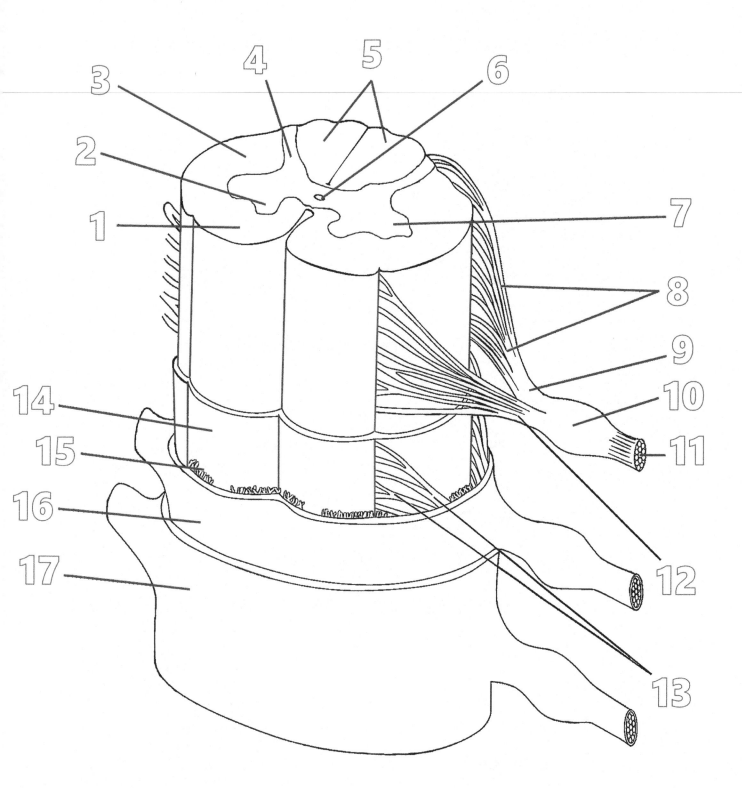

3

4

5

6

2

1

7

8

9

10

11

14

15

16

17

12

13

Color the name and the labeled part:

1. Cerebellar peduncles
2. Superior peduncle
3. Middle peduncle
4. Inferior peduncle
5. Posterolateral Fissure
6. Nodulus
7. Posterior Cerebellar notch
8. Tonsil
9. Flocculus
10. Vermis
11. Fourth Ventricle
12. Intermediate Hemisphere
13. Lateral Hemisphere

The **cerebellum** is responsible for coordinating voluntary movements and functions, including motor skills such as balance and coordination.

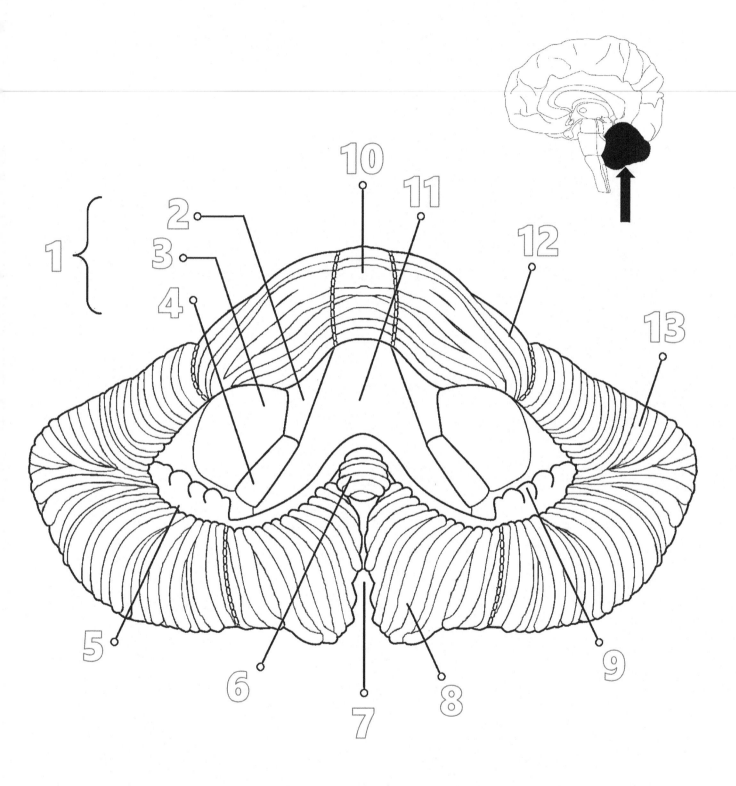

Color the name and the labeled part:

1. Anterior nucleus
2. Ventral anterior nucleus
3. Reticular nucleus
4. Internal medullary lamina
5. Lateral dorsal nucleus
6. Medial dorsal nucleus
7. Intralaminar nuclei
8. Centromedian nucleus
9. Pulvinar
10. Medial geniculate body
11. Lateral geniculate body

The **thalamus** is a small structure within the brain. The main function is to relay motor and sensory signals to the cerebral cortex.

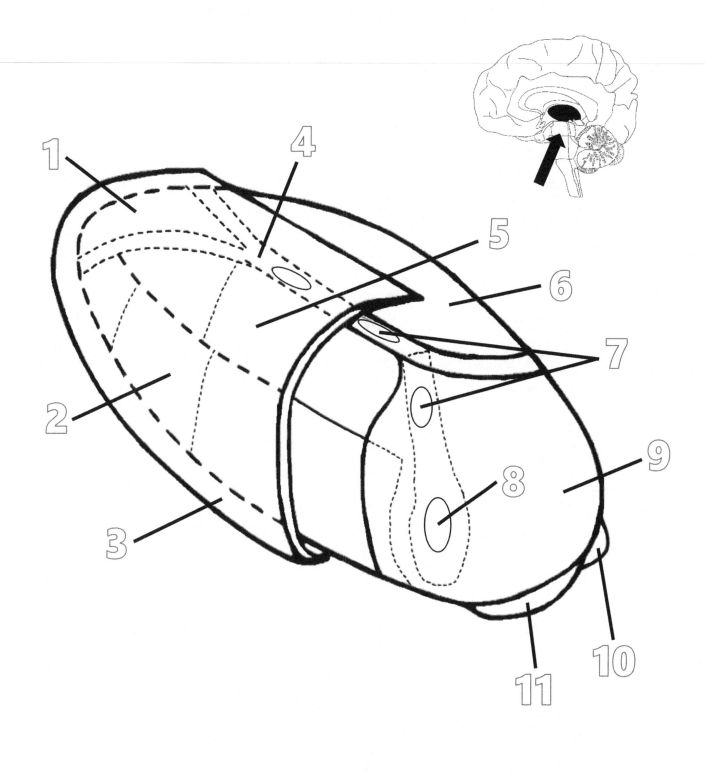

1

4

5

6

7

2

8

9

3

10

11

Color the name and the labeled part:

1. Anterior commisure
2. Paraventricular nucleus
3. Anterior hypothalamic nucleus
4. Preoptic nucleus
5. Supraoptic nucleus
6. Suprachiasmatic nucleus
7. Optic chiasma
8. Fornix
9. Dorsomedial nucleus
10. Posterior hypothalamic nucleus
11. Lateral hypothalamic area
12. Mammillary body
13. Ventromedial nucleus
14. Arcuate nucleus
15. Infundibulum
16. Anterior pituitary
17. Posterior pituitary
18. Pituitary gland

The **hypothalamus** influences functions of regulating body temperature, controlling appetite, regulating emotional responses, and managing of sexual behavior, and controls the pituitary gland. The **pituitary gland** regulates several other hormone glands in the body, including the thyroid and adrenals. The **hypothalamus and the pituitary gland** work together, releasing the correct levels of hormones as the body needed.

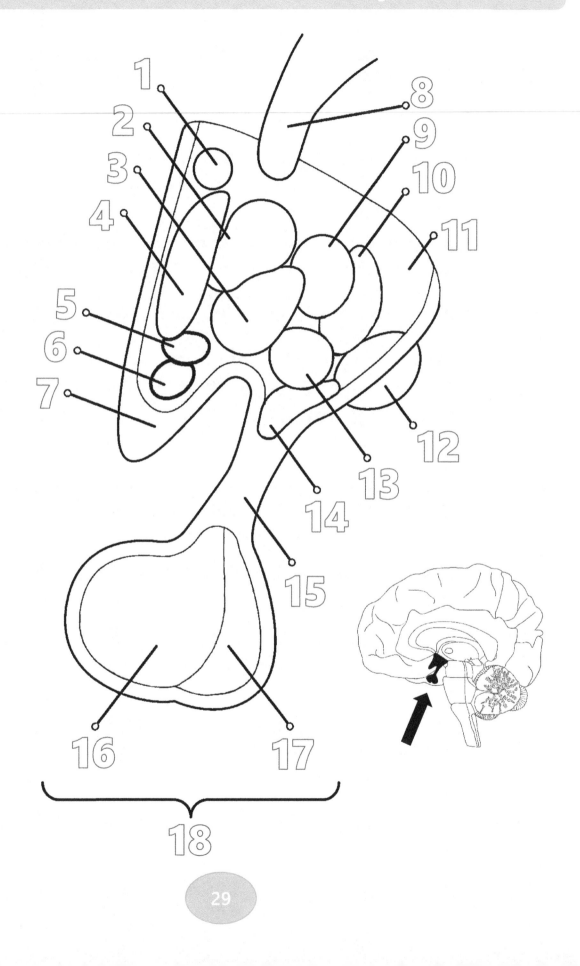

1
2
3
4
5
6
7
8
9
10
11
12
13
14
15
16
17
18

Color the name and the labeled part:

1. **Posterior pituitary hormones**

   - **Antidiuretic hormone - ADH:** It helps to conserve water, prevent dehydration and control the blood fluid and mineral levels in the body.

   - **OXYTOCIN:** It stimulates the release of breast milk, and also stimulates contractions of the uterus during labor.

2. **Anterior pituitary hormones**

   - **Growth hormone – GH:** It regulates growth and physical development. Its principal targets are bones and muscles.

   - **Prolactin – PRL:** It helps the breast to produce milk, and it is secreted in large amounts during pregnancy and breastfeeding.

   - **Thyroid-stimulating hormone – TSH:** It activates the thyroid gland to release its own hormone.

   - **Adrenocorticotropic hormone – ACTH:** It stimulates the adrenal gland to produce and secrete cortisol.

   - **Follicle-stimulating hormone – FSH:** It stimulates the estrogen secretion, and also allows the growth of egg cells in women.

   - **Luteinizing hormone – LH:** It stimulates the testosterone production in men.

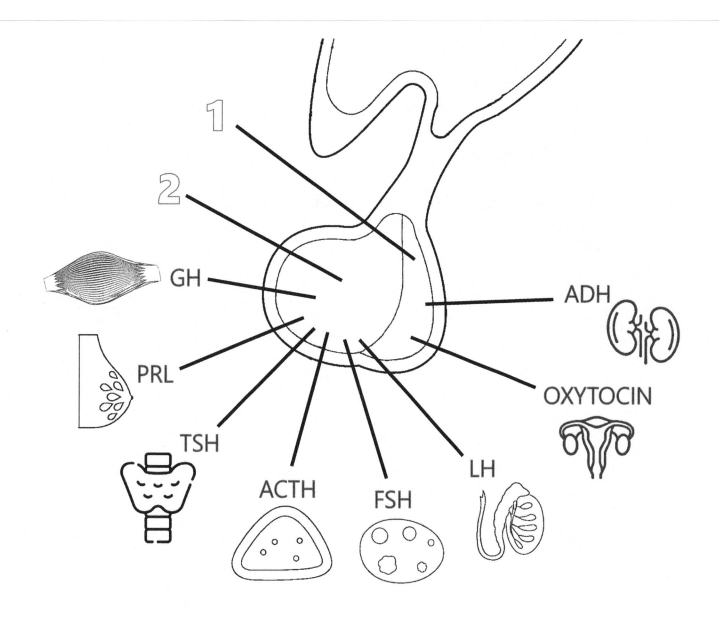

1

2

GH

PRL

TSH

ACTH

FSH

LH

OXYTOCIN

ADH

Color the name and the labeled part:

1. Mammillary body
2. Dentate gyrus
3. Hippocampus
4. Subiculum
5. Hippocampus formation
6. Fornix

The **hippocampus** is a small part of the brain, and it is involved in learning and memory. It plays an important role in the processing of spatial memories, in consolidating memories during sleep, and temporarily storing the information before shipping it off to be stored in long-term memory.

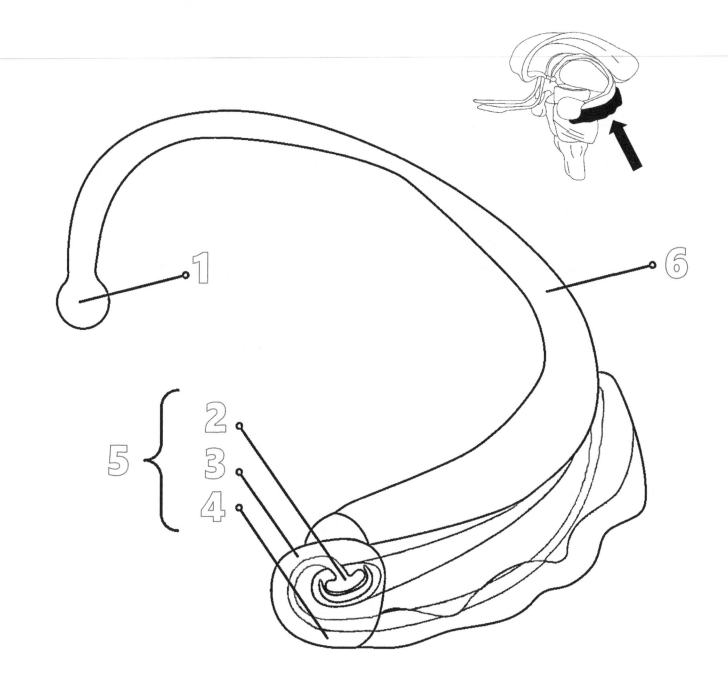

1

6

5 {
2
3
4

33

Color the name and the labeled part:

1. Optic chiasm
2. Optic tract
3. Infundibulum
4. Mammillary body
5. Cerebral crus
6. Pons
7. Middle cerebellar peduncle
8. Pyramid
9. Pyramidal decussation
10. Optic nerve – II
11. Oculomotor nerve – III
12. Trochlear nerve – IV

13. Trigeminal nerve – V
14. Abducens nerve – VI
15. Facial and intermediate nerves – VII
16. Vestibulocochlear nerve – VIII
17. Glossopharyngeal nerve – IX
18. Vagus nerve – X
19. Hypoglossal nerve – XII
20. Accesory nerve – XI
21. Cervical ventral root

The **brainstem** is made up of several components, and they help to regulate breathing, heart rate, blood pressure, and several other important functions.

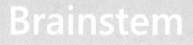

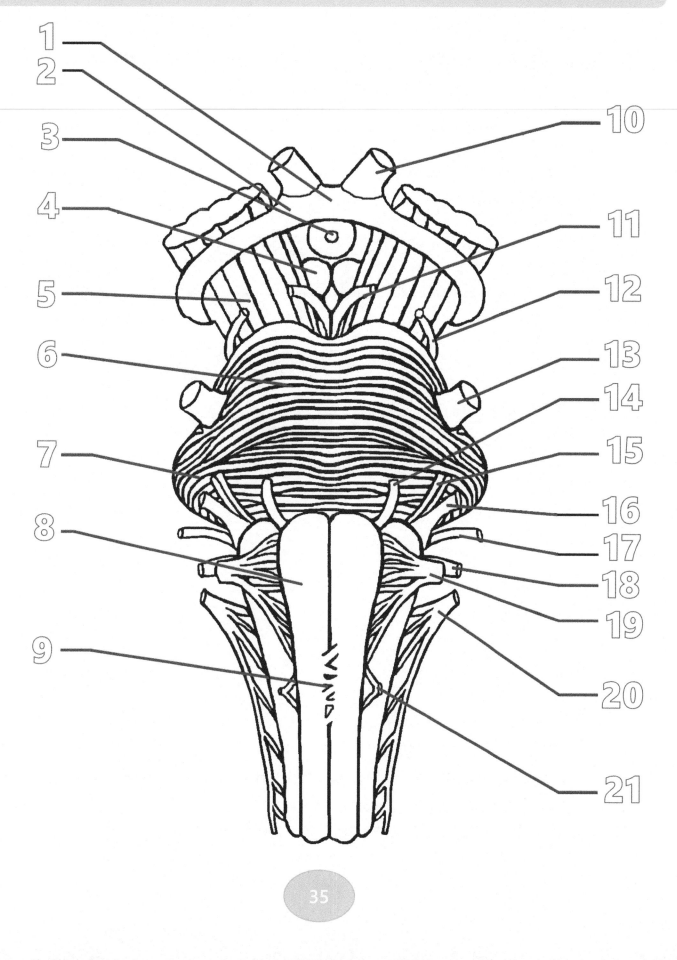

1
2
3
4
5
6
7
8
9

10
11
12
13
14
15
16
17
18
19
20
21

35

Color the name and the labeled part:

1. Superior sagittal sinus
2. Ventricles of the brain
3. Cerebrospinal fluid
4. Arachnoid granulations
5. Subarachnoid space
6. Skull
7. Central canal of the spinal cord
8. Spinal cord

Cerebrospinal fluid is a clear fluid that surrounds the brain and spinal cord, and it cushions them from injury. It is nutrient delivery and is a waste removal system for the brain.

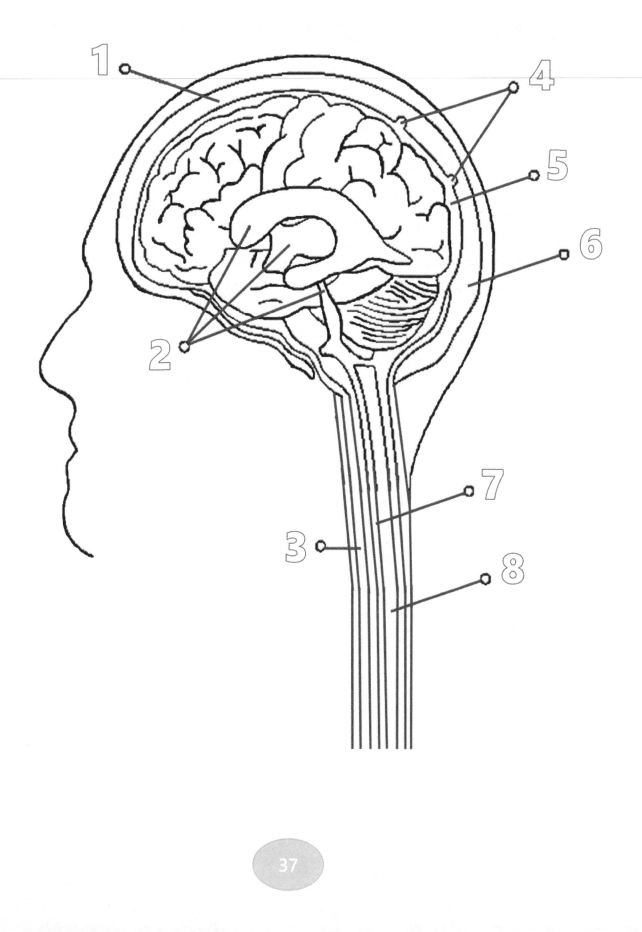

Color the name and the labeled part:

1. Skin
2. Aponeurosis
3. Periosteum
4. Bone
5. Dura mater (meninge)
6. Arachnoid mater (meninge)
7. Pia mater (meninge)

The **meninges** are the membranous coverings of the brain and spinal cord, and provide a supportive framework.

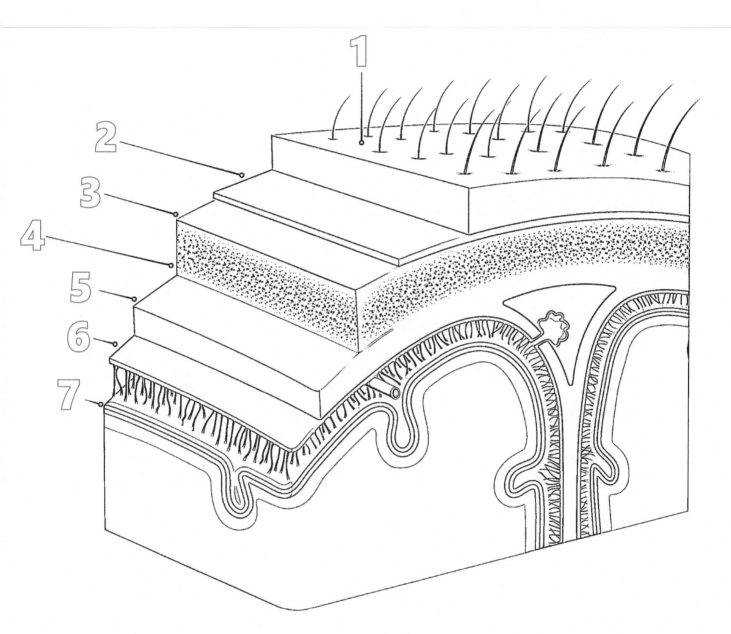

1

2

3

4

5

6

7

Color the name and the labeled part:

1. Fornix
2. Frontal cortex
3. Septum
4. Olfactory bulb
5. Mammillary body
6. Amygdala
7. Cingulate cortex
8. Corpus callosum
9. Thalamus
10. Stria terminalis
11. Hippocampus

The **limbic system** is a set of components in the brain that deal with memory and emotions.

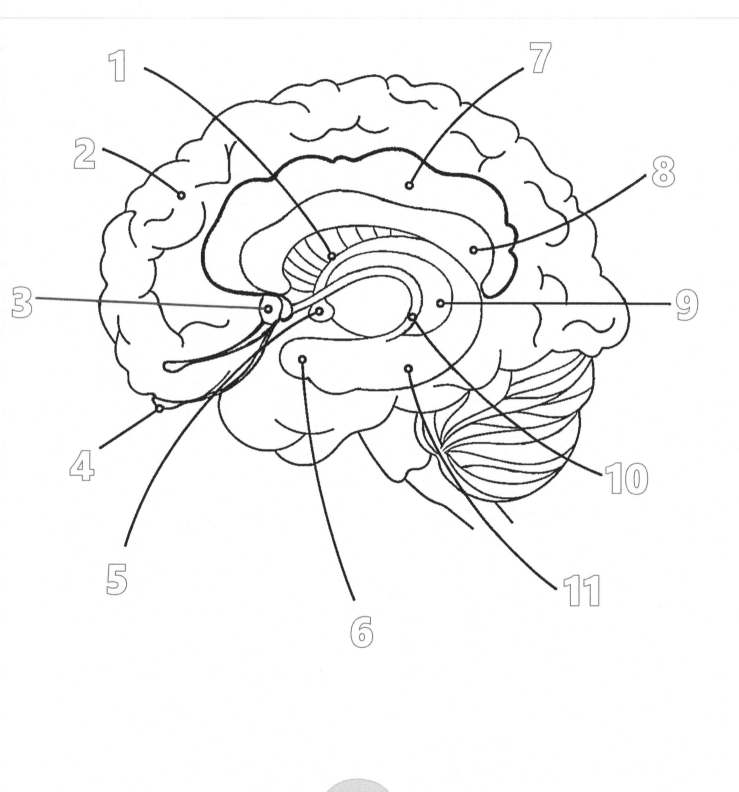

BRAIN FUNCTIONS

- Cerebral cortex areas
- Cerebral lobes
- Cerebral hemispheres

Color the name and the labeled part:

1. Higher mental functions
2. Premotor function area
3. Primary motor function area
4. Primary sensory area
5. Somatic sensory association area
6. Auditory association area
7. Wernicke's area
8. Visual area
9. Memory area
10. Broca's speech area

The **cerebral cortex** is the thin layer of the brain that covers the outer portion of the cerebrum. It is covered by the meninges, and it is gray because nerves in this area lack the insulation that makes most other parts of the brain appear to be white.

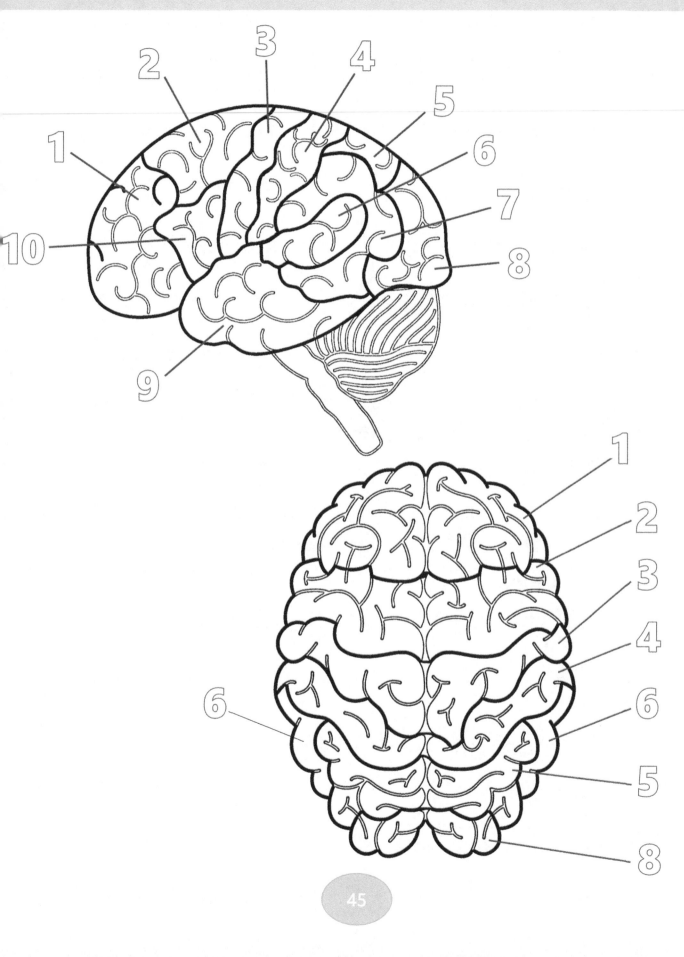

Color the name and the labeled part:

1. Frontal Lobe functions

- Thinking
- Planning
- Emotions
- Motor Function
- Movement
- Short Term Memory
- Language

2. Temporal Lobe functions

- Understanding language
- Memory
- Hearing

3. Parietal Lobe functions

- Sensation
- Reading
- Smell
- Taste
- Touch

4. Occipital Lobe functions

- Vision
- Visual processing
- Color identification

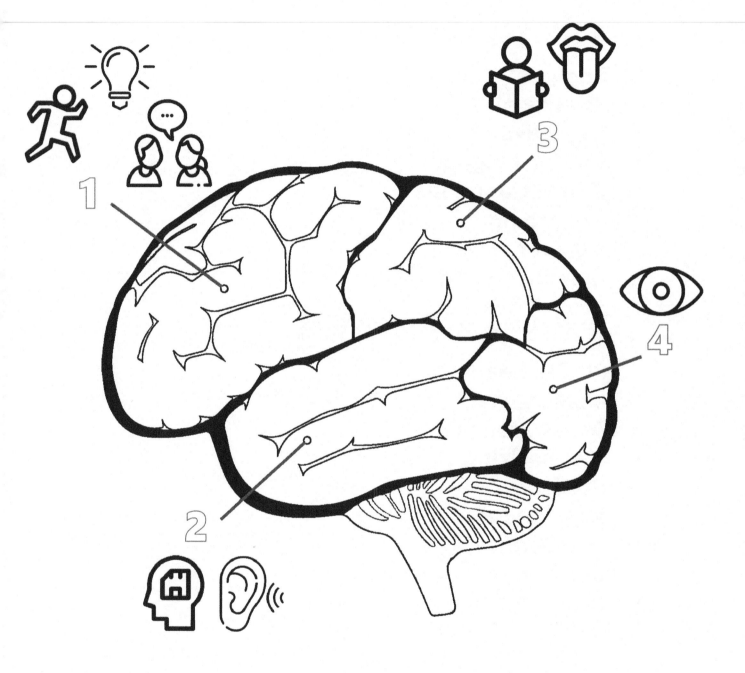

Color the name and the labeled part:

1. Left Brain functions

- Logic
- Analytical
- Objectivity
- Written language
- Spoken language
- Reasoning
- Number skills
- Scientific skills

2. Right Brain functions

- 3D Shapes
- Music skills
- Art awareness
- Synthesizing
- Subjectivity
- Imagination
- Intuition
- Emotion
- Face recognition

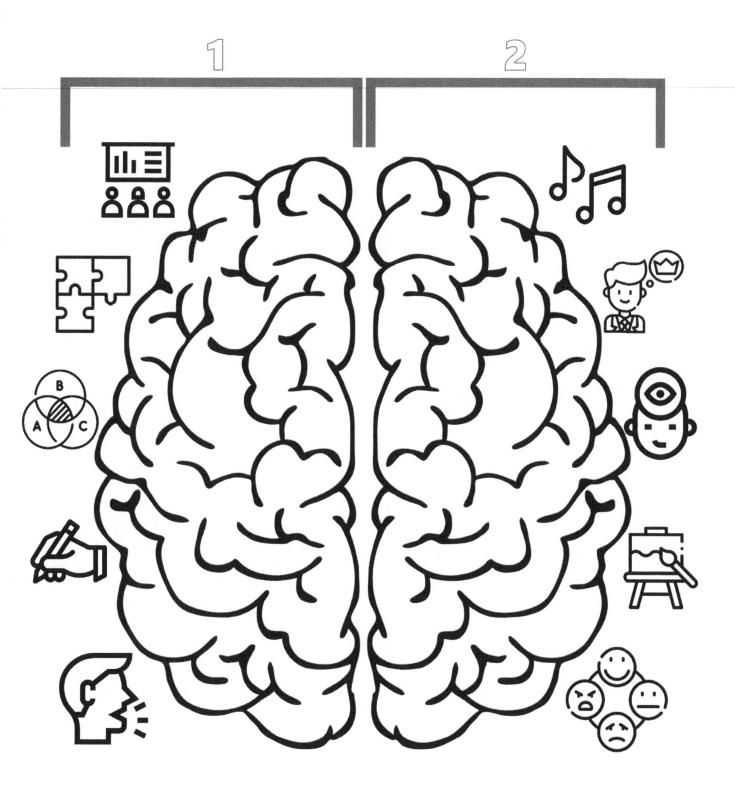

49

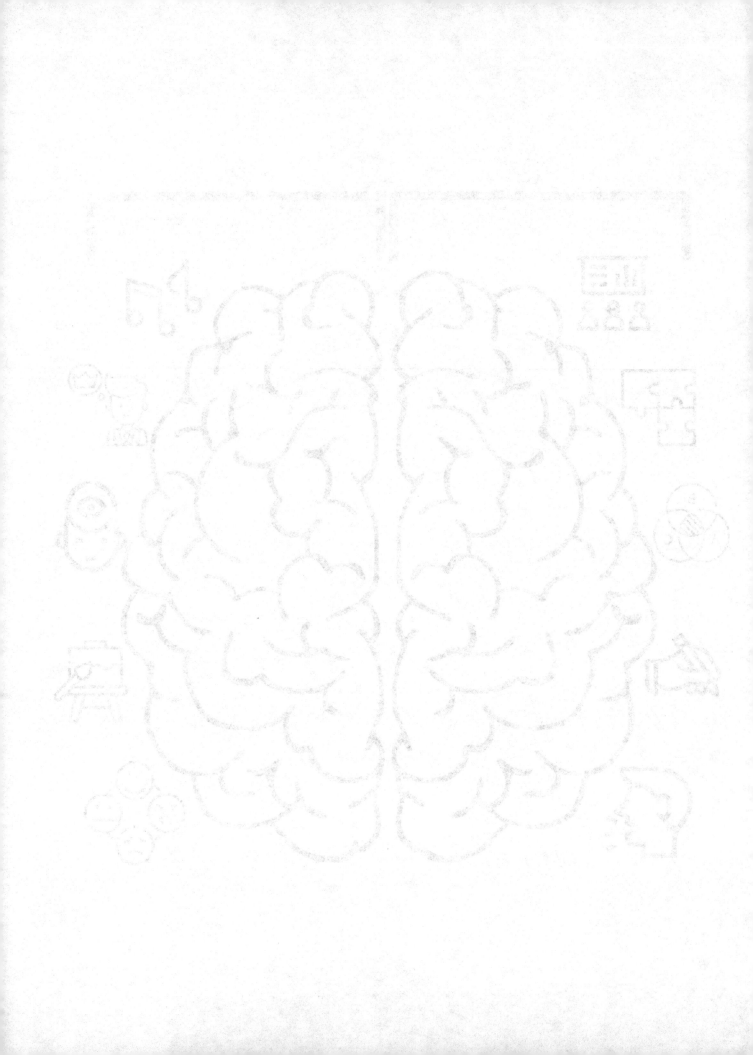

BLOOD SUPPLY OF THE BRAIN

The brain consumes a great amount of the body energy, and requires constant blood supply from the cardiovascular system. That's why, the brain must receive enough blood to function properly.

Color the name and the labeled part:

1. Middle cerebral artery
2. Posterior communicating artery
3. Pontine arteries
4. Anterior communicating artery
5. Internal carotid artery
6. Anterior cerebral artery
7. Ophthalmic artery
8. Anterior choroidal artery
9. Posterior cerebral artery
10. Superior cerebellar artery
11. Basilar artery
12. Anterior inferior cerebellar artery
13. Vertebral artery
14. Anterior spinal artery
15. Posterior inferior cerebellar artery

The **Circle of Willis** is the area where joins several arteries at the inferior side of the brain.

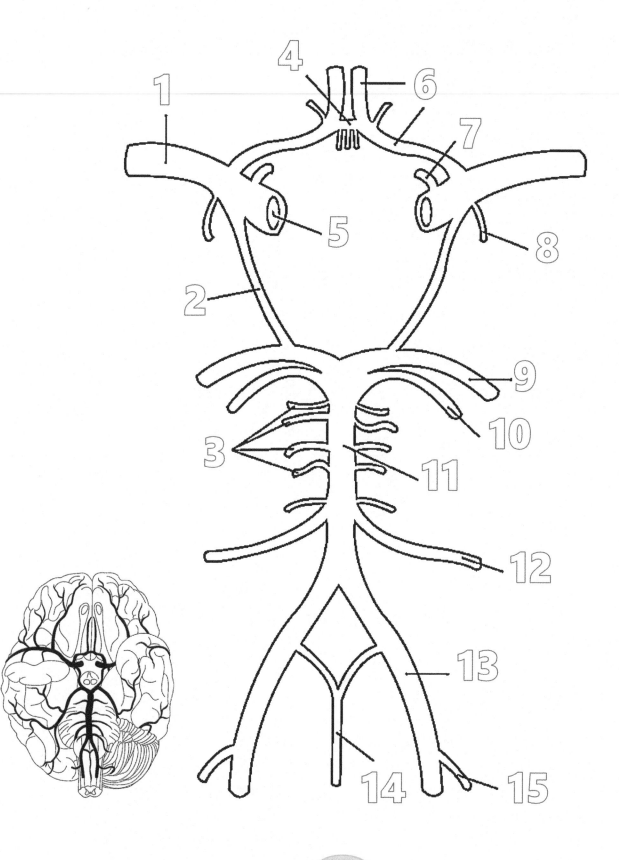

Color the name and the labeled part:

1. Lateral ventricle
2. MCA superior division
3. MCA inferior division
4. Middle cerebral artery (MCA)
5. Internal carotid artery
6. Anterior communicating artery
7. Cerebral cortex
8. Anterolateral central arteries
9. Anterior cerebral artery

The **arteries of the brain** supply the lateral and medial part of the hemispheres, the primary motor area, the sensory language area, the occipital lobe, the frontal lobe, and the superior portion of the parietal lobe.

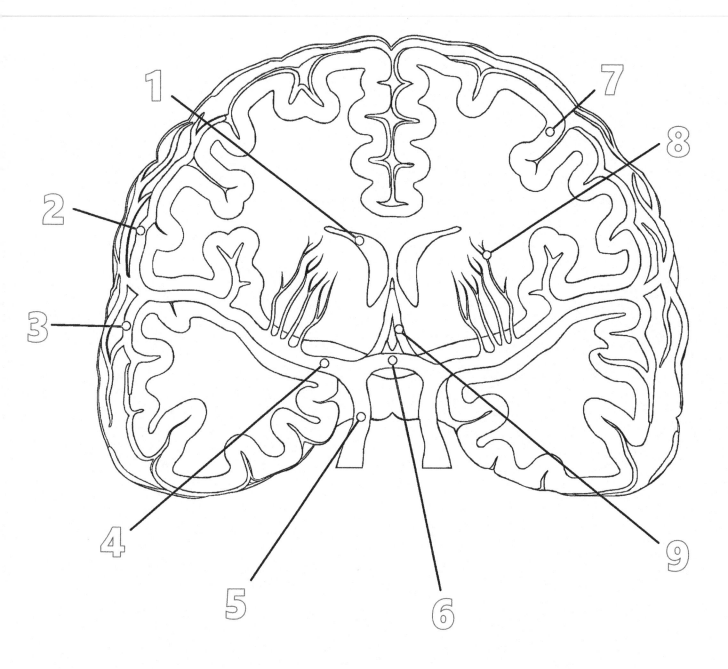

NERVOUS SYSTEM AND NERVES

The **nervous system** is composed by the central and peripheral nervous systems. The central nervous system (CNS) contains the brain and spinal cord, and the peripheral nervous system (PNS) contains the nerves of the body. It is responsible for the consciousness, cognition, behavior and memories.

Color the name and the labeled part:

CNS – Central nervous System

1. Cerebrum
2. Cerebellum
3. Brainstem
4. Spinal cord

Peripheral nervous System

5. Cranial nerves
6. Vagus nerve
7. Intercostal nerves
8. Subcostal nerve
9. Iliohypogastric nerve
10. Ilioinguinal nerve
11. Lateral cutaneous of thigh
12. Genitofemoral nerve
13. Brachial plexus
14. Musculocutaneous nerve
15. Radial nerve
16. Median nerve
17. Ulnar nerve
18. Sacral plexus
19. Sciatic nerve
20. Tibial nerve
21. Common peroneal nerve
22. Deep peroneal nerve
23. Superficial peroneal nerve
24. Sural nerve
25. Pudendal nerve
26. Lumbar plexus
27. Femoral nerve
28. Obturator nerve
29. Muscular branches of femoral nerve
30. Saphenous nerve

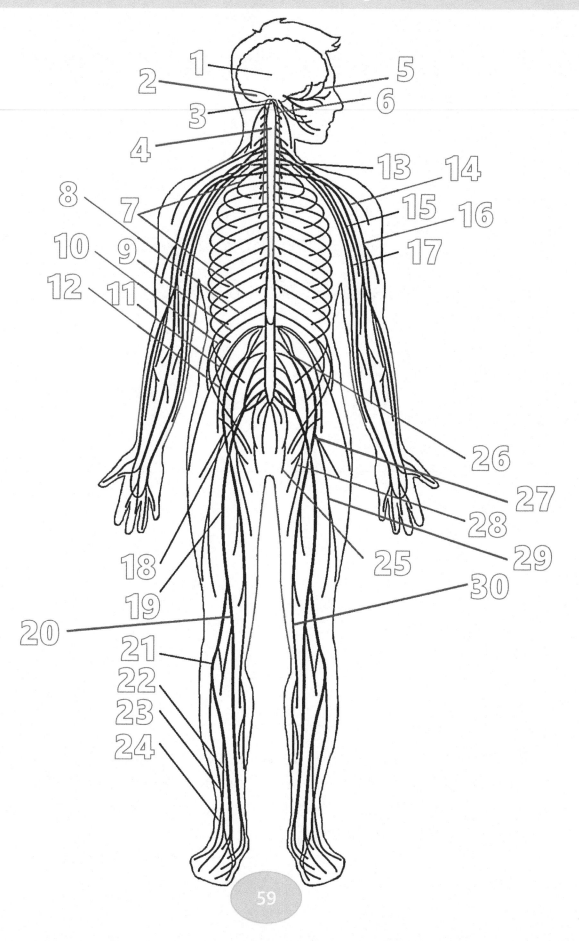

1
2
3
4
5
6
7
8
9
10
11
12
13
14
15
16
17
18
19
20
21
22
23
24
25
26
27
28
29
30

Color the name and the labeled part:

1. Spinal nerve
2. Epineurium
3. Perineurium
4. Unmyelinated nerve fiber
5. Myelinated nerve fiber
6. Fascicle
7. Nerve fibers
8. Endoneurium
9. Blood vessels

ⓘ **Nerves** are part of the nervous system, and are formed by a bundle of fibers which are wrapped around layers of tissue and fat. They are designed to conduct impulses that relay information from one part of the body to another.

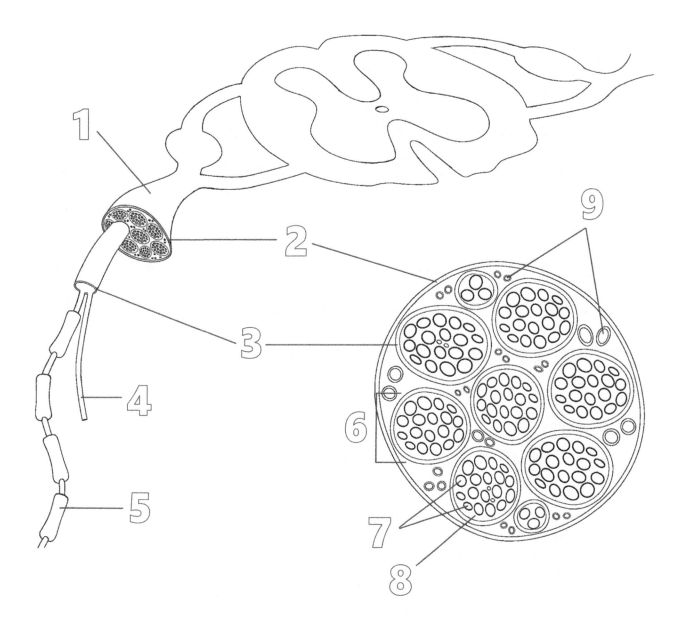

1
2
3
4
5
6
7
8
9

Color the name and the labeled part:

Parasympathetic Nerves Functions

1. Constrict pupils
2. Stimulates salivation
3. Constrict airways
4. Slow heartbeat
5. Stimulate activity of stomach
6. Inhibit release of glucose. Stimulate gallbladder
7. Stimulate activity of intestines
8. Contract bladder
9. Promote erection of genitals

Sympathetic Nerves Functions

10. Dilate pupils
11. Inhibit salivation
12. Relax airways
13. Increase heartbeat
14. Inhibit activity of stomach
15. Stimulate release of glucose. Inhibit gallbladder
16. Inhibit activity of intestines
17. Secrete epinephrine and norepinephrine
18. Relax bladder
19. Promote ejaculation and vaginal contractions

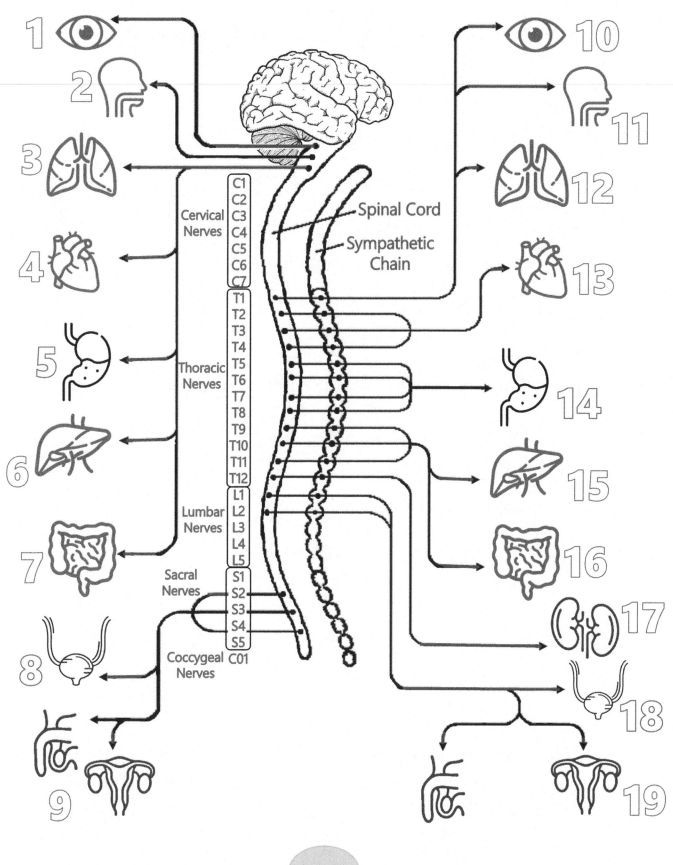

Color the name and the labeled part:

1. Olfactory Nerve - I
2. Optic Nerve - II
3. Oculomotor Nerve - III
4. Trochlear Nerve – IV
5. Trigeminal Nerve – V
6. Abducens Nerve – VI
7. Facial Nerve - VII
8. Vestibulocochlear Nerve – VIII
9. Glossopharyngeal Nerve - IX
10. Vagus Nerve – X
11. Accessory Nerve - XI
12. Hypoglossal Nerve - XII

Cranial nerves emerge from the brain, each one of them is paired and is present on both sides. These twelve pairs of cranial nerves are described with Roman numerals I–XII.

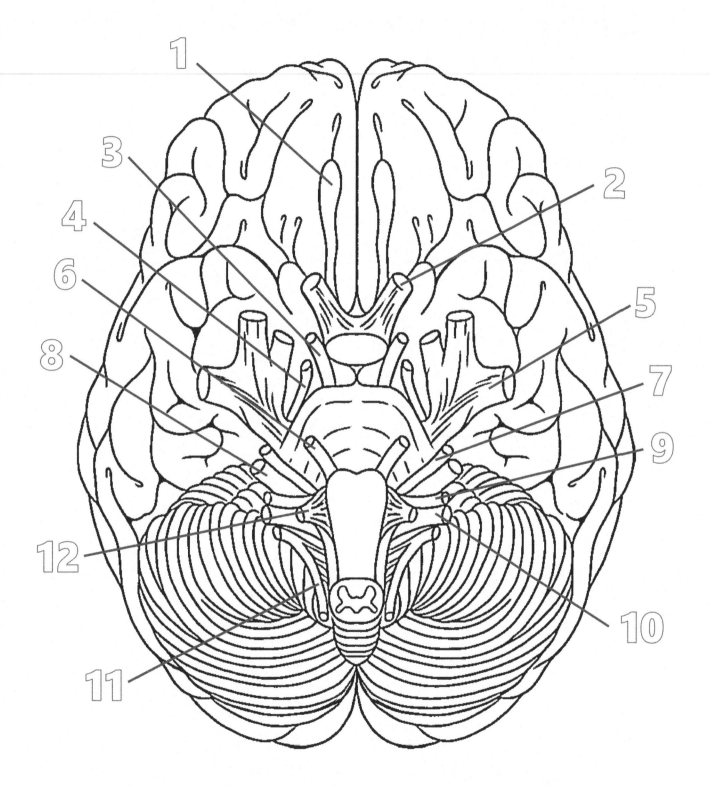

Color the name and the labeled part:

1. Trigeminal nerve ganglion and nuclei
2. Mandibular nerve
3. Ophthalmic nerve
4. Maxillary nerve
5. Superior alveolar nerve
6. Lingual nerve
7. Inferior alveolar nerve

The **trigeminal nerve** is responsible for motor functions such as biting and chewing, and sensation in the face.

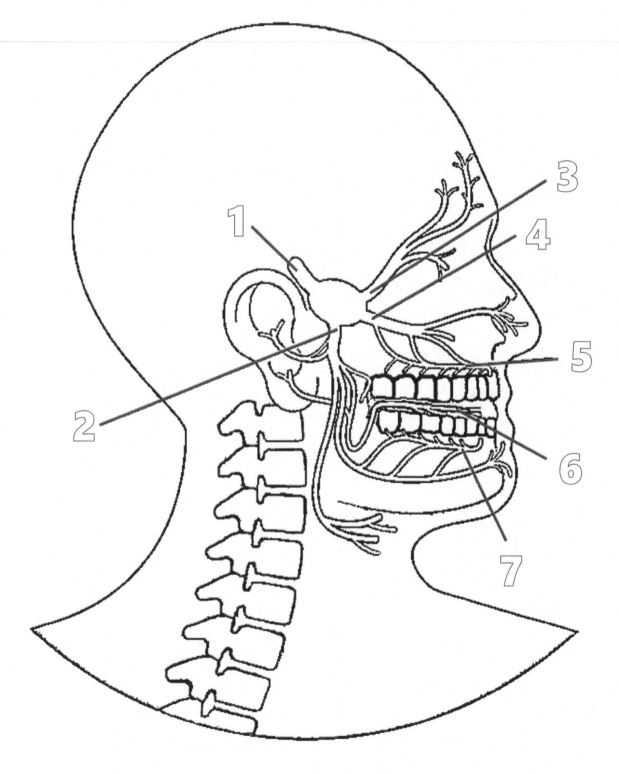

1

3

4

5

2

6

7

Color the name and the labeled part:

1. Vagus nerve
2. Superior ganglion of vagus nerve
3. Inferior ganglion of vagus nerve
4. Pharyngeal branch
5. Laryngeal branches
6. Lungs
7. Cardiac plexus
8. Pulmonary plexus
9. Liver
10. Colon
11. Small intestine
12. Stomach
13. Esophageal plexus
14. Spleen
15. Celiac plexus
16. Kidney

The **vagus nerve** helps with the parasympathetic control of the heart, lungs, and digestive tract.

Vagus Nerve

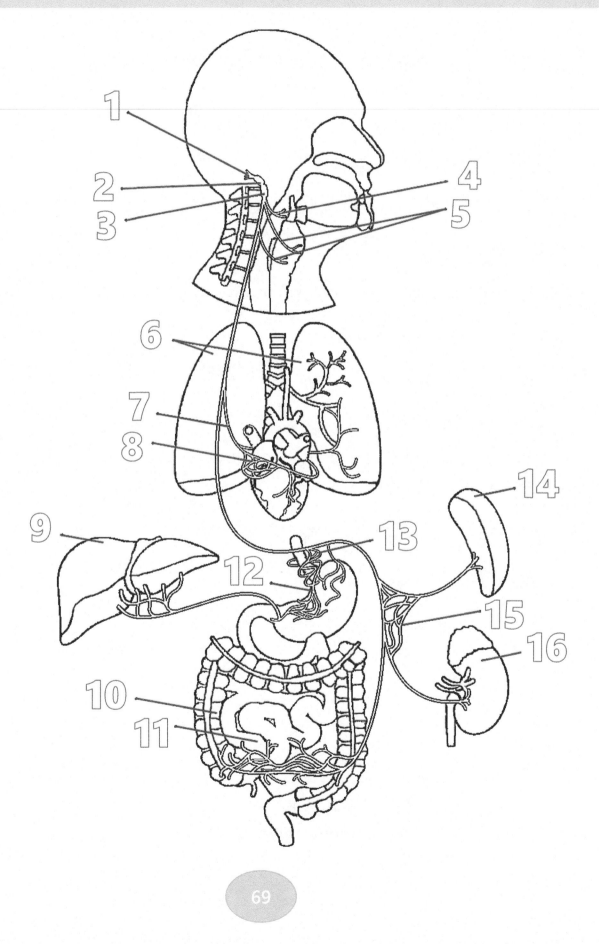

Color the name and the labeled part:

1. Palatoglossus nerve (related to cranial nerve X)
2. Hypoglossal nerve (related to cranial nerve XII)
3. Internal laryngeal nerve (related to cranial nerve X)
4. Glossopharyngeal nerve (related to cranial nerve IX)
5. Lingual nerve (related to cranial nerve V)
6. Chorda tympani nerve (related to cranial nerve VII)

The **nerves of the tongue** help in the following functions: chewing, taste, speech, movement and sense of taste.

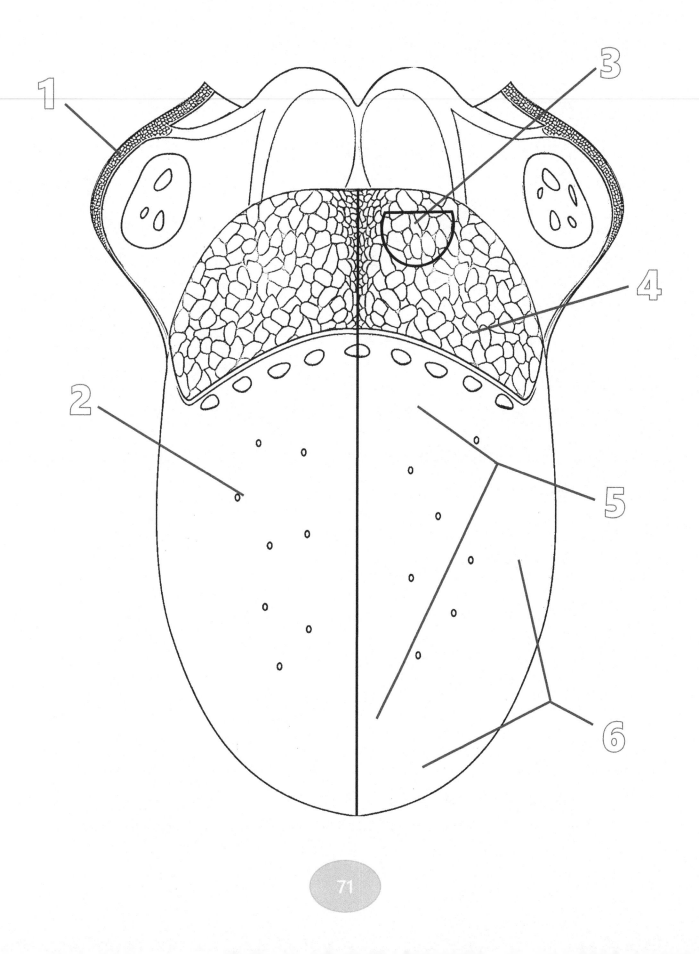

1

2

3

4

5

6

Color the name and the labeled part:

1. Vagus nerve
2. Superior laryngeal nerve
3. Internal branch of superior laryngeal nerve
4. Thyroid cartilage of larynx
5. Thyroid gland
6. Right recurrent laryngeal nerve
7. Epiglottis
8. External laryngeal nerve
9. Superior horn of thyroid cartilage
10. Cricothyroid ligament
11. Cricoid cartilage of larynx
12. Isthmus of thyroid gland
13. Left recurrent laryngeal nerve
14. Trachea

The **nerves of the larynx** control the following tasks: respiration, airway protection, coordination of swallowing, and phonation.

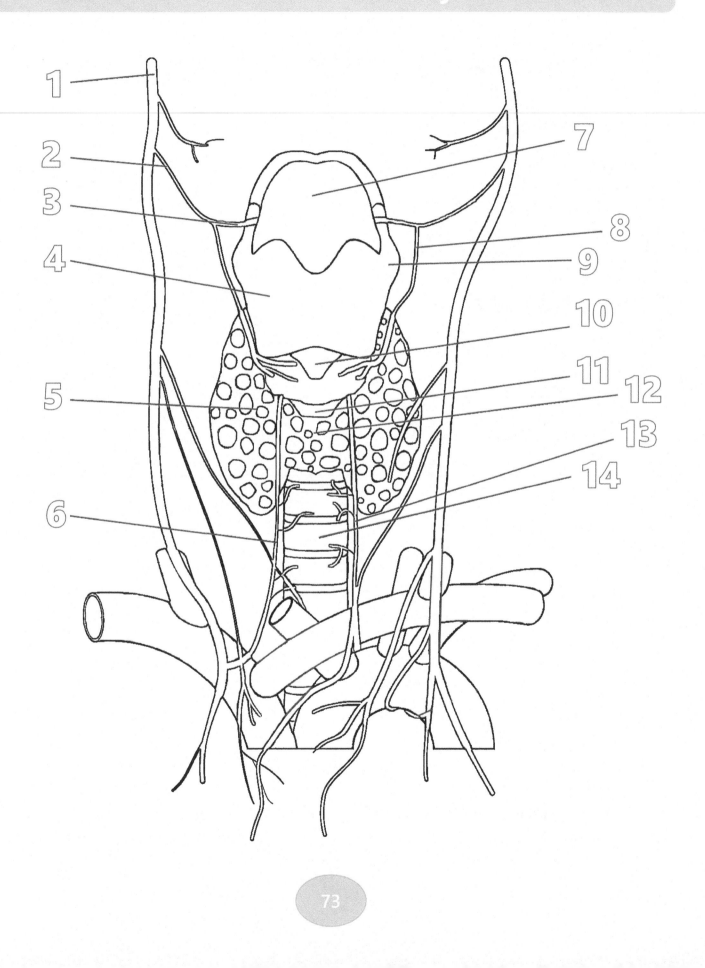

1

2

3

4

5

6

7

8

9

10

11

12

13

14

Color the name and the labeled part:

Arm Nerves
1. Median Nerve
2. Radial Nerve
3. Ulnar Nerve

Hand Nerves
4. Ulnar Nerve
5. Median Nerve
6. Radial Nerve

The **nerves of the arm and hand** are part of the brachial plexus. They control the muscles of the shoulder, arm, forearm and hand.

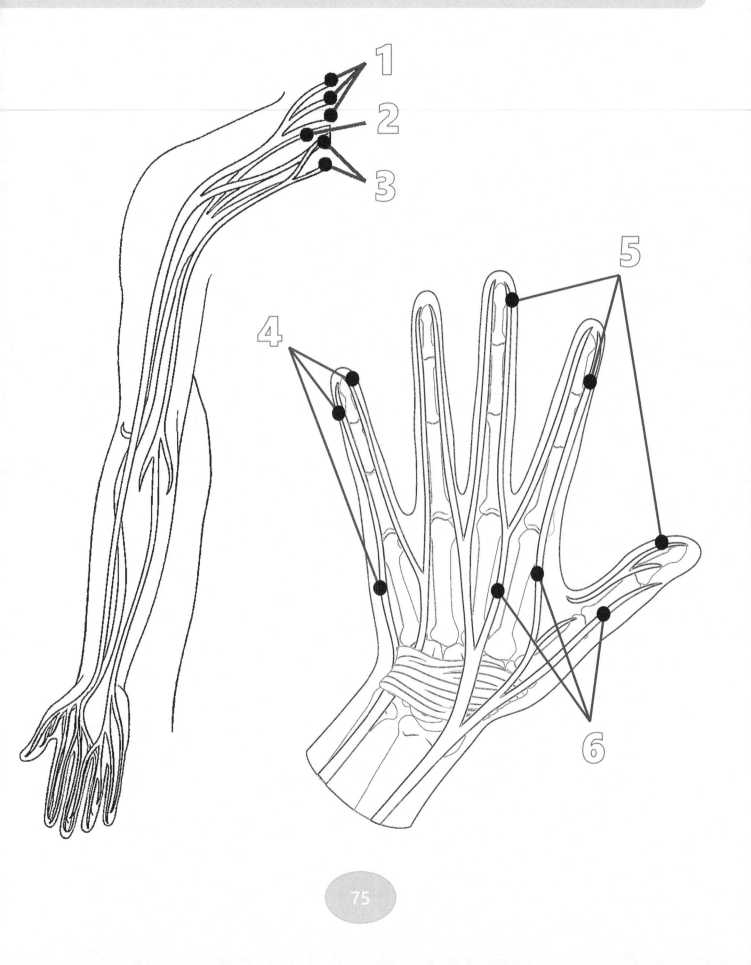

1

2

3

4

5

6

NEURONS

The **neuron** is the fundamental working unit of the brain, that send and receive signals to other nerve cells, such as other neurons, muscles, and glands.

Color the name and the labeled part:

1. Soma
2. Nucleus
3. Dendrite
4. Schwann cell
5. Node of Ranvier
6. Myelin
7. Axon
8. Axon terminal

A **neuron** is formed by dendrites, an axon, and a cell body or soma.

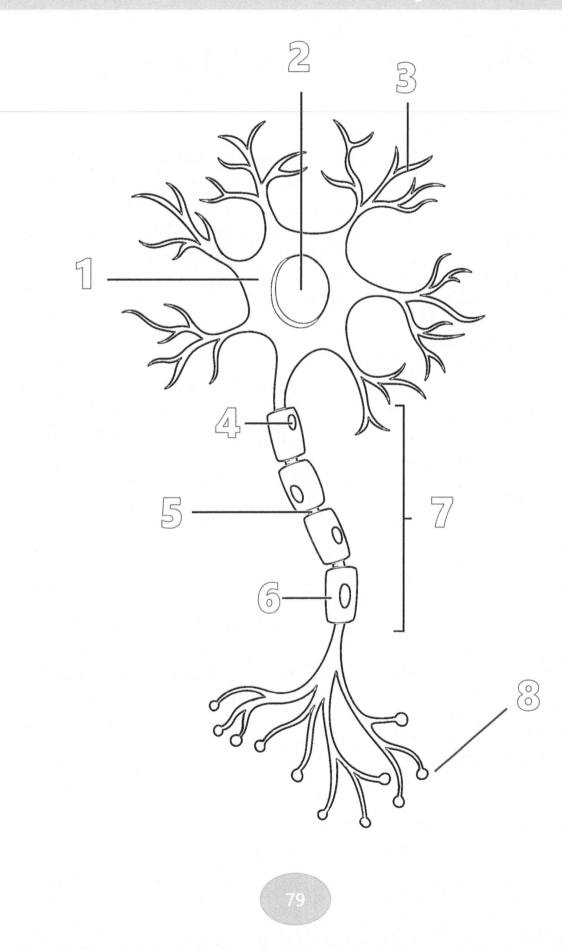

Color the name and the labeled part:

Sensory Neuron

1. Myelin
2. Nucleus
3. Axon
4. Axon terminal

A **sensory neuron** is a nerve cell that receives external signals from the environment, and transmits the information in the form of electrical impulses.

Motor Neuron

1. Myelin
3. Axon
4. Axon terminal
5. Dendrite

A **motor neuron** is located in the motor cortex, brainstem or the spinal cord, to control organs, muscles and glands.

Interneuron

1. Myelin
3. Axon
4. Axon terminal
5. Dendrite
6. Cell body

An **interneuron** has an integration task, and helps to connect and transfer signals between sensory and motor neurons.

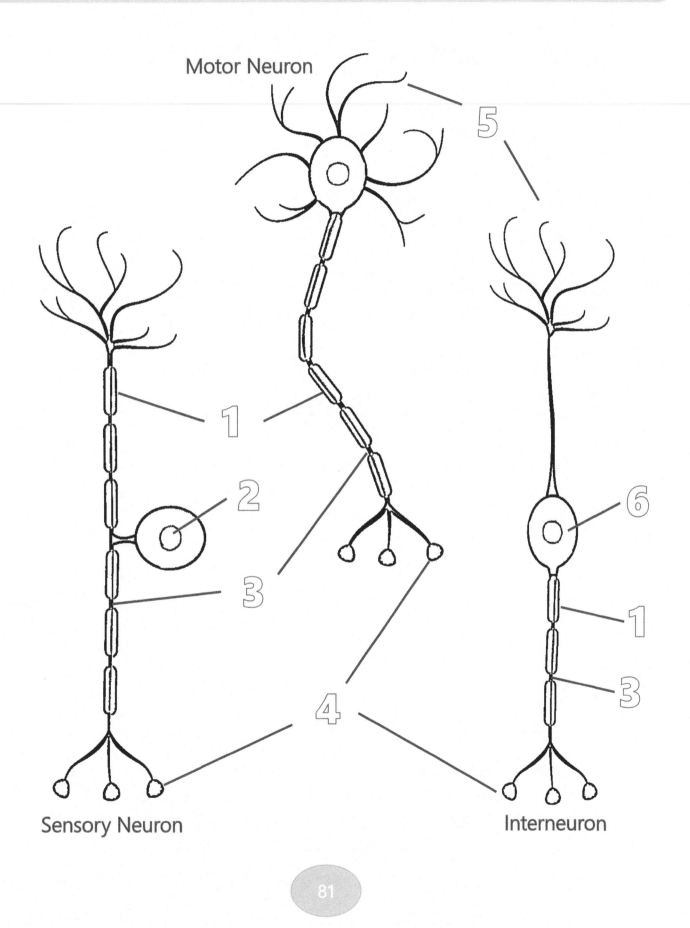

Motor Neuron

Sensory Neuron

Interneuron

Color the name and the labeled part:

1. Nucleus
2. Dendrites
3. Myelin sheath
4. Axon
5. Axon terminals
6. Muscle cell nucleus
7. Muscle fiber
8. Neuromuscular junction

A **motor neuron** connects muscles, glands and organs of the body, sending information from the spinal cord to skeletal and smooth muscles, and regulating all muscle movements.

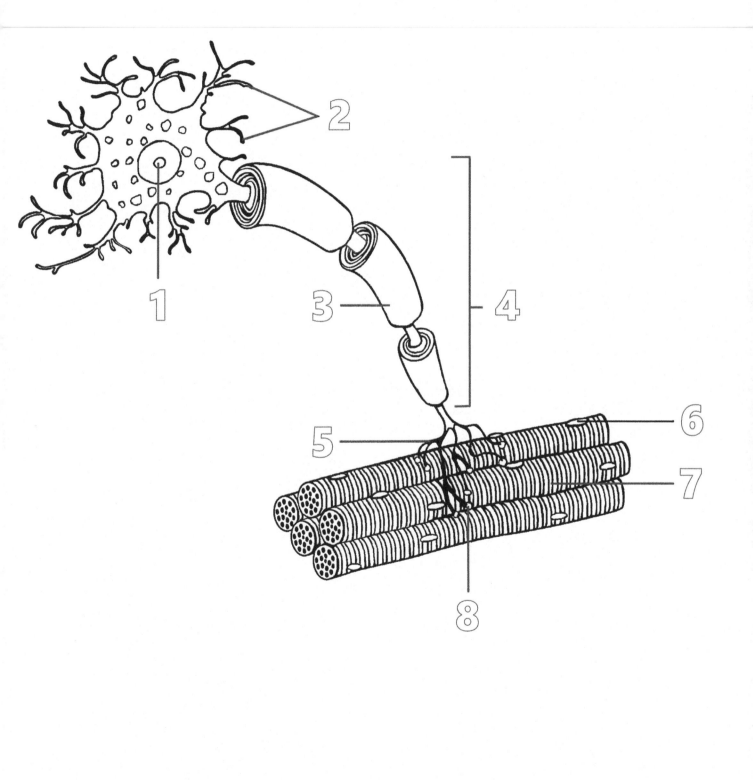

CONCLUSION

Thank you so much for your purchase, and I would like to tell you that I am very happy to help you learn the basis terminology about the neuroanatomy.

If you enjoyed this book, then please leave an Amazon review. Reviews are the lifeblood of our publishing endeavors- leaving a review would mean the world to us.

Thanks again!

Summer Q. S. Parks
TFC Guide Publishing

Available now on Amazon

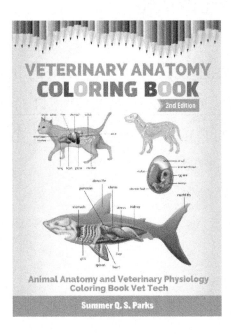

★★★★★

PAPERBACK ASIN: B08JVR5MH6

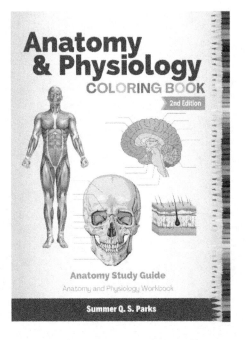

★★★★★

PAPERBACK ASIN: B08P1B4W1M

JUST A QUICK FAVOR...

Please you feel free to send us any comment or suggestion through the next channels:

Email: admin@tfcguide.com

Please write me by email and I will send you digital templates as a gift.

Our goal is to improve and create more valuable books for you.

Thanks again!

Summer Q. S. Parks
TFC Guide Publishing

ACKNOWLEDGEMENTS

I would also like to thank the valuable contribution of these people who inspired the creation of this book:

- Patrick J. Lynch, medical illustrator. For the next illustrations: Ventral view of the Brain and Cranial Nerves (Permission = Creative Commons Attribution 2.5 License 2006)

Thanks again!

Summer Q. S. Parks
TFC Guide Publishing

More books by
Summer Q. S. Parks

SCAN ME

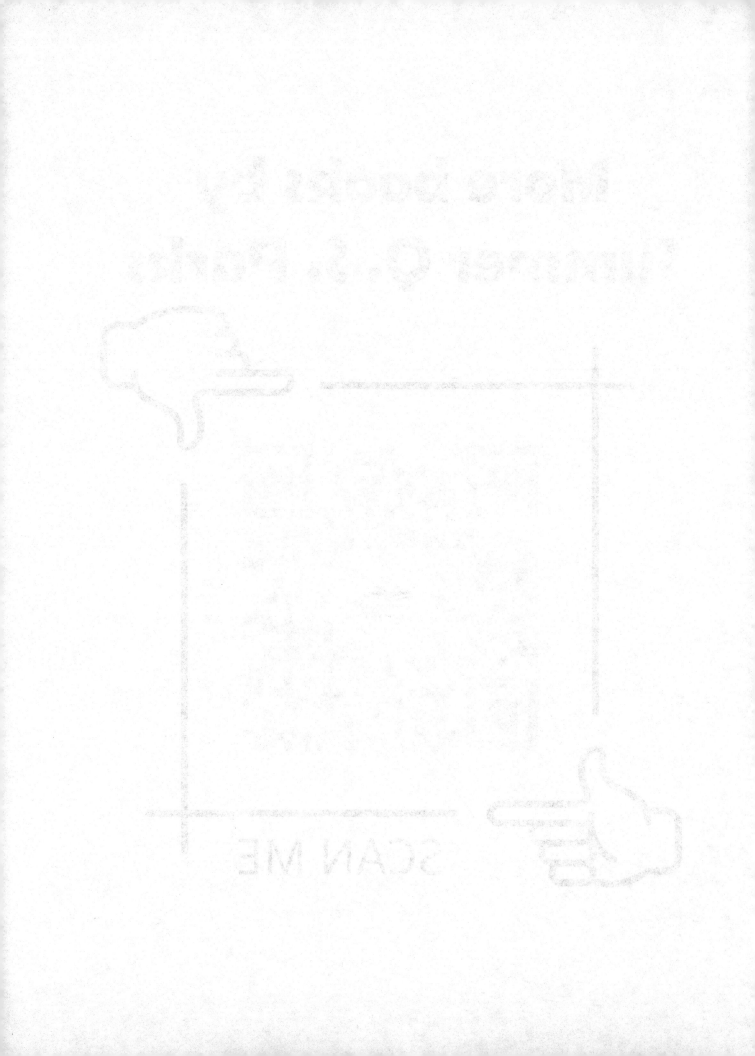

Made in the USA
Monee, IL
03 January 2024

51076238R00052